*You Are the*
# PATIENT,
# I Am Your
# NURSE

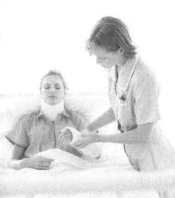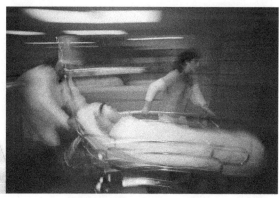

## SUSANLEE WISOTZKEY
**PhD, BA, BSN, RN, NE-BC, HNB-BC, PLNC**
**Alumnus CCRN**

PAGE PUBLISHING, INC.
Conneaut Lake, PA

First originally published by Page Publishing 2020

ISBN 978-1-6624-1418-3 (pbk)
ISBN 978-1-6624-1419-0 (digital)

Printed in the United States of America

# DEDICATION

I write this for my family, my brother, my sister, my father, my mother, and all my patients whom I have had the privilege to serve.

I hope to give you a glimpse of the heart of nursing or the absolute selflessness needed to be unbiased and see past the exterior to be there with you, for you, your advocate.

A special dedication to my sister,
Amy, whose profound emotional depth can be
found in the poetry contained within.
May the angels give you and brother Joe wings to soar.
May your heart find the peace you search for.
May you both rest in peace.

## The Dandelions

*In patches of soft gold and green,*
*The meadows are a lovely scene.*
*The gentle feel of misty dew*
*Will cling to me and clean me through.*
*The morning sun does slowly rise,*
*And underneath the golden skies,*
*I'll run through meadows soft and green*
*And fill my soul with golden sheen.*

*—AW*

# PROLOGUE

Every day someone asks, "Why do you do what you do?"

I have decided you, my patient, should understand the reason behind the why.

Every weekday, weekend, holiday, every day, I am here for you.

During the day, in the evening, and all night long, I am here for you.

I am always near to ease your pain, answer your questions, or be a sounding board for your anger, frustration, and loss of control, guilt, or sadness.

I endure the wrath of your family, your spouse, your children, and your physicians. I still come back each day to be with you, my patient.

Why?

My head is tired, my feet ache, and my heart is heavy at the end of each day. Yet tomorrow I will be back to work, by your side with a smile and a shoulder to lean on, because you are my patient. And maybe, just maybe, I can give you a day with a little less pain or a little more caring; maybe you will even smile, just once.

Even if you do not smile, even if you abuse me, throw things, or are just downright mean, I will return tomorrow.

Why?

*Because you are my patient and I am* your *nurse.*

## Page Duex

*Emotions are not me;*
*I am they,*
*Though they were made to be*
*A good way*
*To communicate,*
*But a counterweight*
*Must be found*
*To expound*
*Them to another*
*As a brother*
*Or of love.*

*—AW*

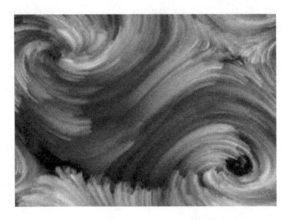

*Shared from the writings of Amy Ellen Wisotzkey Martorell (AW)*

# CHAPTER 1

My name is Susan; I want to be a nurse.

The year was 1961. I was five years old, and you were my older brother. I idolized you. You were my hero, my companion, my best friend. The sun was shining brightly, and we were climbing the mounds of dirt created by the bulldozers building the house next door to Aunt Jess. We were laughing, taunting one another, and daring the other to do more extreme stunts. You started a sprint from the top of the dirt mountain, stumbled, and fell headfirst. You slid almost to the very bottom of the dirt mountain. Everything seemed to go into slow motion. I can still hear your scream, filled with agony and pain, piercing my ears and my heart.

The blood was gushing down your leg from the long cut just below your knee. You cried so loud; I felt so helpless and so sad. I made you get up, and together, we hobbled back to Aunt Jess. I just knew we needed her. She is a nurse. She would know what to do to make you better. All I wanted was to see you smile, your big, grinning, carefree smile, one more time.

I was young, yet I stayed with you while Aunt Jess effectively and efficiently cleansed and mended the long gash just below your knee. Your eyes sparkled through the moistness left by your tears. I believed I had just witnessed an angel perform a miracle. Your smile was as big and bright as I remembered.

I knew at that very moment, my destiny was to be an angel too.

The years passed quickly. I am six, seven, eight, and I was a roller-skating princess. I skated at the local rink twice a week for practice and on Saturdays for fun. I competed for speed in my age group. I am a competitive winner. I am fast and fearless. I was petite, maybe four feet, six inches, weighing about seventy pounds. I trust everyone, which translates to "I am friendly without alarm." I have long blond hair and bright-green eyes.

One day I was helping with handing out rental skates on a Saturday afternoon. As I walked to the back to get a drink of water, strong arms surrounded me from behind, one around my waist, one covering my mouth, lifting me off the floor. I could not scream. This old man ran his hands all over my body I struggled and fought until I could break away. I do not really recall how old he was. I was young, and anyone my parent's age or above, I thought of as old.

My sparkle dissolved into gray; now I knew fear. I was so small, so young. Why would someone do that? I never returned to the skating rink. I did not have the ability to fully digest or comprehend the ramifications of what happened. I just knew I did not want to go there anymore.

Ten, eleven, I was stronger now; my fear replaced with stubbornness. I listened to the stories told by my friends and their siblings. I said nothing, but I realized I am not alone. This was a revelation that gave me an inner strength that grew exponentially.

I was almost a teenager when I came home from school to find blood trailing through the open back door. Why was the door open? I cautiously entered, following the trail through the family room down the hall into the kitchen. My head was spinning. There was blood splattered everywhere. I slipped in the pool on the floor. I looked up and saw droplets on the ceiling. As I stood up, there were blood streaks across the counters, clots that look like sections of liver in the sink.

I did not scream. I did not faint. I was curious and frightened. My mind flew through a burst of questions: What happened? Who is hurt? And how can I help? Upon continued investigation of this horrific scene, I saw a blood-spattered note neatly set next to the stainless steel sink:

Went to hospital. Be home soon.

Love,
Mom

Now I panicked inside. What do I do? I knew my brothers and sister would be arriving home from school soon, so I cleaned the kitchen and took care of my siblings until my mother returned.

An hour or so later, it seemed like an eternity. Mom came through the door in a whirl with a huge bandage around her hand. What, when, where, how—all questions were flying out of everyone's mouth. Mom had severed the tip of her finger completely off with the hedge cutters, and they sewed it back on. *Wow!* I was fascinated; my siblings thought it was disgusting. It looked like it was sewn on as if one would tack stitch the hem of a skirt with *X*'s. The miracle of medicine, I was hooked.

I had direction, purpose, desire, and commitment. I was on my way; I was going to be an angel (like Aunt Jess) in the field of medicine (like the people who sew fingers back together).

Twelve, thirteen, fourteen, I was a candy striper (a volunteer) in a local hospital. I had never been so happy. I loved the medicinal smells, the excitement and energy of all the grown-ups, the way they could make a sad patient smile and give hope to families and children all at the same time.

Fifteen, sixteen, a laboratory technician took me under her wing and taught me more than I could have imagined about the human body from the inside out. Urinalysis, parasitology, blood counts, microbiology—my mind was a sponge, soaking in every bit of knowledge. It was summer; I was now a trained phlebotomist and planning for senior year in high school. I loved life. I loved work. I was going to be a nurse.

It was now the end of summer. I was sixteen when my life was turned upside down and went sideways.

Everything changed, never to be the same. The little boy with the cut on his knee, my brother, was in a crippling motorcycle acci-

SUSANLEE WISOTZKEY

dent. He was the passenger and catapulted headfirst into a large tree. The tree won.

I was working at the hospital when the trauma tones pierced the silent hallway. "Trauma Emergency Department" flashed on the screen. I was clueless. My pager started beeping. I was the hospital float phlebotomist, covering the ED and stat labs on all seven floors of the hospital. I knew the moment I walked into ED trauma. My colleague grabbed my right arm and forced me out of the room. I spun around because of the hold she had on me. There in front of me I saw my mother sobbing. The hospital chaplain gently cupped her elbow, guiding her to a quiet room. I quietly followed. Once in the room, I gazed at pictures on the walls. Eventually, my eyes landed on my father, who sat motionless, as if a statue staring into nothingness.

Joe passed without regaining consciousness—a motorcycle accident, massive head trauma, and a severe brain injury, with brain stem herniation. There was no hope; medicine had not risen to the level to care for such a devastating injury.

The sadness was overwhelming, deep, and suffocating. My air was gone, my inner light was flickering, and my heart ached under the weight of the sorrow filling my soul.

I watched his lifeless body on that cold steel-framed stretcher covered by a white sheet. I saw and recognized his feet as he vanished from my sight forever—a sight forever etched in my mind. I wanted to scream. I wanted to go bring him back. I was frozen. My colleagues rallied and told me to go home.

I was thinking, *Why would I go home?*

I went for a long drive to all the outdoor places we would go together with our friends. I exited my car. Top of the world—that is what we called this place. I sat down and cried for a very long time.

How does one cope?

Where does a person start? How do I start over? What does that mean?

How do I just go on?

Funny thing is, you do just move along because time does not stop. My friends did not speak to me. They avoided me. They were so sad. They had no words. They were afraid. Death was now real to them. They did not know what to say, so they said nothing. I was alone.

My family, my home, my brother and sister were alien to me. We barely spoke. We essentially coexisted in a mutual space. There were no words or actions to change to result.

*Lonely souls in a immense void.*

I needed to get out of there. I needed to find the joy in life again. My focus intensified. I knew what I needed to do—continue on my course and help others who face traumatic incidences—and people need to know they are not alone, not forgotten. We all need hope, faith, and some assistance through personal tragedies, someone to assist, someone to listen, to provide guidance, resources, connections, if appropriate to a path or plan to regain control over one's life, one's destiny.

## Arising

My emotions explode into bits, dangling on the edge of my mind,
Dripping into pools of hazy tranquility,
reflecting scenes of past and future.
I feel a tightening within me,
Them a reaching of my mind into dimensions
of color, causing a reality of unreality.
Then blackness encircles me, and a kind of peace reigns within my soul.
Now electric streaks of pain spin out of me.
I hear the wailing of a thousand souls.
O Lord, have mercy upon me,
For I fear this land into which my soul has wandered.

I walk into the light again,
The dawning of a new day.
Peace and tranquility reign in this place.
Silence cloaks it in mystery.
The sea before me shimmers in golden light of the rising sun,
While the birds' melodic tweets greet this glorious day.
Angels descend from the heavens,
Carrying souls away,
Forever.

—AW

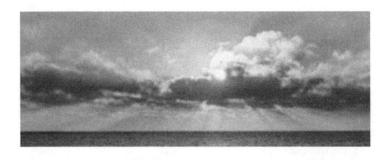

# CHAPTER 2

I left high school at the age of sixteen, graduating a year early and attending the local college as a freshman. I was sad to leave my friends and all the social activities of senior year. I knew in my heart, my decision was the best choice under the current circumstances. I could sense my friends were uncomfortable around me. They did not know how to deal with death, sadness, or anyone that reminded them of the inevitable consequence of life. I was that reminder to them; they could not deal with me. There were only unspoken words and sullen eyes of silence. I was alone.

My family structure slowly disintegrated; my parents divorced, and my youngest sibling was shipped to a private school in another state. I moved to northern New Jersey to continue to follow my dream.

I was a junior in college, ready to start my senior year. I felt invincible. I was a somewhat reckless teen, invincible, and I was eighteen.

The rain was falling; it was dusk, a few sprinkles mixed with fog as I cruised down the highway, pushing eighty miles an hour. I was homeward-bound and anxious to see my family. Lightning flashed; my world went black. I felt cold liquid running down my face, my dark silence interrupted by someone yelling. I did not understand the words. The lights were too bright. I could not breathe. The darkness folded around me like a cloak as I disappeared into the abyss.

Time passed, an unknown amount of time. I opened my eyes to see I was in the hospital, my hospital, my chest fractured and my ankle crushed. The doctor bluntly informed me, "Your ankle fracture may have severed the artery. We will watch it closely, but you may lose your foot. We will do what we can. Best-case scenario, your ankle will be frozen and you will have a limp." Then he said I was very lucky. Who says this to a teenager? Then he turned and walked away.

Lucky? Ha, what is lucky about this? What happened? Where is your compassion? Where is my family? What is happening? This cannot be real. As denial set in, I drifted back into darkness.

My life was ruined. Every dream, aspiration, miracle was gone in the blink of an eye; I remembered a flash of lightning. Maybe this was a dream, a terrible, horrible dream. I will just close my eyes, and when I wake up, everything will be all right. It was not; I was living my nightmare.

My hospital course was extraordinary; I met a young man (I will call him Gary) who lost his leg in a traumatic accident on a farm. When we met, he was learning to walk with a prosthesis. I met young woman (I will call her Sally) who refused to participate in her recovery, refused to even try, and denied that she was in worse shape than I was. Sally had a broken back and numbness in both legs.

The challenge was on.

The young man, Gary, was twentysomething, with sandy hair and bright-blue eyes that twinkled when he laughed. He laughed a lot. Leg or no leg, he was determined to be whole. I liked his positivity. We schemed, planned, and made Sally our project. He joked with her and eventually broke through her tough exterior. They did not realize how much they helped me. *Remember when I was ten. I learned the power of strength in numbers. Humans need one another.* Together we all began to heal, from the soul level to the physical level, each of us going our separate ways when the time was right.

I returned to the university the following fall for my senior year. I graduated at the age of nineteen, but not in nursing. My fractured ankle and crutches kept me from my required clinical rotation. It was not my time to be a nurse, yet. Apparently, there were many more lessons on the horizon for me to learn.

*Life is a journey of lessons learned.*

# CHAPTER 3

My name is Susan; I was a new bride, but I wanted desperately to be a nurse.

Nineteen, a whirlwind year, I married my college sweetheart, lived on a horse farm, and had no idea what adulthood was all about. It did not take long for reality to set in. And it hit really hard.

I went to work as physical therapy assistant; my husband stayed at home and partied with his friends.

Soon, he was working too, but our lives were already beginning to show different paths. We stayed together for several years; we had a son, a beautiful, smart, incredible son.

Even though we did not last and our marriage dissolved, our son had been the focus of both of our lives and set the precedence for our continued friendship.

*You cannot undo that which has been done.*

My path led me back to the local hospital as a nursing assistant. I enrolled in the vocational school, licensed practical nurse program. I attended LPN training and then applied for loans to continue my education to become a registered nurse.

Then the final straw, the last stressor that destroyed our marriage…the phone rang.

"I have some bad news," the voice said. The voice was not familiar, yet I knew they wanted to talk to me. I felt the sadness before I heard the words.

"Your sister suffered a traumatic injury. She passed away a few minutes ago." I later found out she suffered from a gunshot wound to the head.

My younger sister's body was flown back from Texas. She was laid to rest beside our brother.

May their souls rest in peace.

This was a challenging time for both my son and me. I was working full-time, raising a child, and now a single mother attending college. I was a licensed practical nurse.

I was tired.

My motto: *"Patience is a virtue."* I was twenty-five.

## *Presence*

*Black, silent night, wraps me in warm, moist caresses.*
*In silver silhouette, you dance through dappled forests,*
*Chasing each other into the fields. The moon's bright light*
*Reveals them to the white phantoms. Watch and move*
*And live as one, 'til dawn's drenching dew*
*Casts asunder their bond of warmth, and they wake*
*Into the different worlds their eyes can now see,*
*Each turning toward their final destiny.*

*Then I shall wake on the white shore of an azure sea*
*To watch the sun splinter amethyst and rose across the water.*
*Sea spray and wind upon my face, with the bitter taste of salt*
*Upon my lips, while the sand grows hot beneath my feet.*
*And forever, I shall not cherish any tomorrow*
*More or regret any yesterday.*

*—AW*

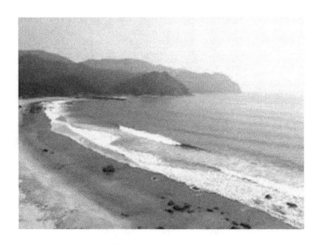

# CHAPTER 4

My name is Susan; I am a nurse.

Twenty-six, I am a registered nurse in an intensive care unit. I know so little, and I know so much. It is incredible. I am here.

*Life has a way of throwing curveballs.*

My last, my only sibling is missing. His first-floor apartment trashed, everything turned over, emptied onto the floors in every room. Yet his motorcycle is there, on the porch, locked, undisturbed, as if all is well. All the doors are hanging open. He is nowhere, gone, just…gone. No one has heard from him in days.

Days turn to weeks, weeks to months, months to years, and no word, no sign. He has just vanished.

Fear grips my soul. What if…I never see him again? I am down.

*I feel the echoes of loneliness from the past, the silent whispers in my mind.*

My patient arrives direct from surgery. No time to dwell on the past, maybes, or what-ifs. The patient comes first, *always*.

The surgeon is asking for suction. The anesthesiologist is asking for the respiratory therapist and the ventilator. We need medication for the blood pressure, *now*.

We are a team working in a synchronistic motion, everything accomplished in a few moments of time. The patient is settled in, equipment with its rhythmic swish, blood pressure under control. Patient has stabilized, but there is a long night shift ahead. A lot of work to do to maintain that stability.

I am a night nurse in the open-heart intensive care unit.

My patient is seventeen years old. Status: post open-heart surgery.

I now understand the phraseology "You are very lucky." This young adult presents with a fence post through his chest.

A big post! A really *big* post!

He lost control going around a curve. His car went off the road—*bump, bump, bump*—down an incline and through a fence. The fence is composed of thick wooded posts and electric wire, to keep cattle from crossing. The car sheared off one post, catapulting it through the windshield, piercing Tommy's chest, and anchoring him to the front seat.

Medicine has come a long way in the past twenty years. Tommy arrived in trauma bay with the fence post intact. Immediately he is prepped and rushed to the operating room. No time to waste. Our golden hour is closing. The open-heart team is standing by. Surgery continued through day shift and evening. Tommy arrived to open-heart intensive care, sometime after 2:00 a.m. I am the night nurse in OHICU. Tommy is my patient.

Youth has its merits, especially in the body's innate ability to heal. The course of treatment was uneventful. By day three, he is extubated, eating, and ready for his first walk around the unit.

Miracles are stories of strength, hope, faith, and resilience, which continue to be both amazing and intriguing.

I love being a nurse. I am making a difference, *one patient at a time.*

*My heart is a desert,*
*Void of all feeling but the lonely call of the wind and sand.*
*And in this desert, nothing grows, for there is no rain.*
*And the heat of the sun burns a hole right*
*through my soul, and there is pain.*
*I have learned much, but the wisdom is so hard*
*to come by that I wish to learn no more.*
*I reach to God for help, but there is no answer, so I have put*
*all my thoughts, my feelings, my very soul on paper.*
*And through time, my heartache may be cured.*
*For time, the great healer of all, shall carry my words to become*
*the past, and perhaps the future holds better things.*
*My heart is a desert,*
*Void of all feeling but the lonely, sad call of the wind and sand.*
*But someday my summer shower shall come and, with it, life and love.*
*And flowers shall bloom.*
*My day will come when the desert is turned to meadow, rich and fertile.*
*I await the day.*

*—AW*

*I await the wisdom of experience and time.*

# CHAPTER 5

## Tina

*The day was bright and fabulous; the sky slowly churned through shades of gray, as the snow began to gently fall and then continued for hours. The snowfall increased, creating whiteout conditions. As the snowfall slowed to an eventual stop, the accumulated snow glistened with shades of blue and pure white under the light of the full moon. On this evening, after the snowfall tapered off, Tina and her friends decided to venture out on an adventure.*

*For privacy's sake, I will call her Tina. She is sixteen years old. Her friends say she is pretty. She is not too tall, a little "busty" for her age. Her hair is blond and falls in soft curls to her midback. Friends and family say she loves to push to the limit. I am sure she makes her mother crazy with worry.*

*Out she went on this extraordinary evening on a fabulous adventure into the wondrous snow-covered world, Tina and her friends. The moon was beaming, full in all its glory. The snow sparkled like diamonds under the moonlight. They drove out into the countryside, where they decided to see just what the car could master. The driver, though too only sixteen, had a good driving record and was skilled as a driver. He intentionally spun the car. The excitement was incredible. After several passes and several spins, Tina popped open the sunroof and stood on the seat. "The sight was glorious, the snow sparkling around me like stars fallen from the heavens above. As we went into the spin, I was on top of*

*the world. Like a princess I was, with my long flowing diamond-studded*
*white dress spinning around me.*
   *"Something went terribly wrong. I was cold, so very cold, and the*
*pain was intolerable... Sirens, I think...*
   *"I hear sirens, and then dark oblivion surrounded my being."*
   *(This is from a note. she wrote to me during her hospitalization.)*
   "Tina, Tina," I said. She opened her beautiful sky-blue eyes. She
was intubated and unable to speak. I took her hand. "Tina, you are in
the ICU. You are my patient, and I am *your* nurse." She began to cry,
no sound, just tears quietly rolling down her milky-white cheeks. She
closed her fear-filled eyes and was still. The medication was helping
to keep her comfortable.
   Tina had multiple crash injuries, including her chest and pelvis.
Her light-blond hair appeared to have streaks of orange from the
blood that had trickled through it. Days passed, and Tina continued
to improve; her anxiety lessened. We spent many hours together. I
would hold her hand and just quietly be there. Other times, I took
great care in combing out the tangles and knots in her long hair.
With each day, Tina lay in her ICU bed; the tangles increased and
began to clump into matted knots. Each day I would sit with her and
comb out the knots as we communicated in our way, me verbally and
Tina writing notes.
   Finally, the day came, and Tina was extubated. Together we
rejoiced, and she gave her aunt permission to cut her hair into a
"short bob" just below her chin.
   Tina's improvement was short-lived. Complications set in
quickly within two days as fibrous tissue began to grow in her lungs.
She was re-intubated, her eyes so sad, tears dripping from the cor-
ners. Hours turned to days—no improvement. Yet each day I would
care for her, as I would want someone to care for my child. The physicians spoke at length with the family. I sat with Tina and explained
our plan for transfer, why, when, and how. I told her everything I
could think of to make the transition as smooth as possible. I hugged
her before her transfer. Her heart was pounding and her breath more
labored even on the ventilator. My prayers went with her.

Tina returned to our ICU a week later. She smiled around her breathing tube. Her color had improved. There was a sparkle in her eye. I took report on her condition, potential problems, implications, and warning signs. Three days passed. Tina never complained, was no longer demanding, though she did like company. It was subtle, the change. Tina would slowly clench her hands into fists when I would say I would be back. Her eyes opened a little wider. She was afraid to be alone. This was different. Yes, this was a change, and not for the best. The trauma physician called. He came to the unit immediately, orders written and carried out, my fear and suspicion confirmed.

The fibrotic tissue was continuing to grow and now was invading both lungs.

I entered Tina's room; what I witnessed surprised me. There was a change in her eyes, a knowing without boundaries. I saw the expanding wisdom in her eyes. Her gaze was straight and steady, eye to eye with me. I knew she knew.

She reached out for me. I gently held her hand and sat by her side. She knew; I do not know how, but she knew. I could not speak. My throat felt like it closed, as if my heart leaped up and was blocking off all sound. I just shook my head slowly back and forth. Tina let go of my hand and scribbled on her notepad: "I'm all right. It's okay." She was not afraid anymore; she seemed very peaceful and calm.

*You are my patient, and I am your nurse.*

*And sometimes, we learn to let go.*

Tina transferred, once again, to the university hospital. It was snowing that night, a gentle flurry, and the air was cool as it filled my lungs. I said a prayer and wished her well on her journey.

Tina never came home.

I think of her often, especially when the moon is full and shining across the newly driven snow, sparkling like stars that fell from the heavens, or "a flowing diamond-studded white dress" reaching over the continuum of time: past, present, and future.

My patients touch my heart and my soul. Life is precious.

*Pain inside me, like flames, licking the sides of a hollow bowl,*
*Shooting in and about me like blades of grass*
*shooting up under warm summer suns.*
*This pain makes my mind like fog along the seashore, thick and cold,*
*Reaching through my veins, into the tips of my fingers,*
*widening, to fill the very air that surrounds me.*
*It shoots from my very skin like tiny sparks of static*
*electricity, to form a pattern of dancing lights.*
*It weaves around my heart like thread on a*
*loom and slowly in creeps within.*
*It fills my soul, and like unto rainwater, its*
*clarity, so crystal, is almost beautiful.*
*And now the pain dies quickly, as do leaves in the autumn.*
*It falls away as the tide from the shore, only to come back again,*
*As forever as the sea and the sun, as lonely as the dead.*
*But I welcome it for its loneliness may conquer mine.*

*—AW*

# CHAPTER 6

## *Mac*

It has been a long week, trauma after trauma rolling through the ICU doors. I was finally looking forward to a day off. One more night shift to go. I arrived early to the unit for my shift; I sat down to discuss my assignment for the night. I had only one patient. He was small, only five years old. His prognosis was not favorable. One shift, I wanted to cry.

He was so small, so innocent.

Earlier in the day, Mac was a ball of fire, no limit to his energy. He ran and played and ran some more. He loved his new swing set with the big sliding board. Up the ladder and down the slide, round and round he would run, down the slide and around and up the ladder. She said she only looked away for a moment. When she looked back, where was he?

She ran out to find Mac hanging caught between the swing set support and the slide. He was cyanotic, blue. Unresponsive, he was not moving. Desperation and courage gave her, his mother, the strength to get him unwedged and down. With her cell phone, she called 911. She recalled it seemed like hours of CPR, the sirens so far away. Would they find them in the backyard? She prayed, all the while doing CPR on her lifeless, limp child.

I met Mac that night. Intubated, quiet, and eerily still. The only movement, the rise and fall of his chest as the air pushed into his lungs by the ventilator. I introduced myself to Mac and his father. I explained the nursing plan of care for the shift.

The silence was deafening. Dad just sat there in the chair, staring at his little boy.

I started my assessment, speaking softly and explaining every touch and movement to Mac. His little face was speckled with petechia, a tiny purplish red spot on the skin caused by the release into the skin of a very small quantity of blood from a capillary. This is a sign of strangulation injury.

I knew in my head this was not a favorable sign, but my heart stayed positive and strong. In between physical care, I sat and spoke, softly telling Mac stories. Dad asked why, stating, *"He can't hear you."*

I explained that hearing is our last sense and many patients, when they awaken, remember things that were said to them or from others talking in the room. At first, Dad was skeptical, but he joined me in telling Mac stories. He emphasized about how important it was for him to get better, that he was the most important person in the world to his mom and dad.

Just being there was ripping my heart out. As my shift came to a close, Mac moved his left hand. I thought Dad was going to have a stroke. Then Mac's dad yelled. I thought I would have a stroke with him right there, right now.

I was not sure at first; I did not want to get his hopes up. This movement might have been reflexive. I performed a standard mini neurological exam, equal, round and reactive pupils, cough and gag reflex intact, withdrawal to minimal noxious stimuli. Then the true test… "Mac, squeeze my hand," I said in a quiet voice next to his tiny ear. He did, very weakly, but he held on. Reflexive, maybe. "Mac, now let go." He did as requested! I told Mac's dad I would be right back. He stared blankly at me. I was elated.

I called the trauma physician.

He was already in the ICU seeing another patient and came over to Mac's room. He, too, was skeptical. He gave me "that look." After his examination, he smiled. I felt my heart swell with joy. The doctor explained the findings to Mac's dad, careful not to give too much hope. We still did not know if there would be neurological impairment secondary to the anoxia (lack of oxygen to the brain).

I was cautious with my words to the father and continued to care for Mac just as I had all night. As I ended my shift, Dad asked if I would be back. I told him I was scheduled off. Tears filled his eyes. *"Please come back. Mac needs you."*

My name is Susan. I *am* Mac's nurse.

I agreed to work the following open night shift.

When I returned, the following evening, Mac was weaned from the ventilator. This is a process that takes time and patience, small steps. Bit by bit, the team of doctors, nurses, respiratory therapists, and of course, Mac's dad (who was there all night) successfully removed Mac's breathing tube by morning's first light. Examinations and evaluations one after another, trauma, neurology, and pediatric specialists. The results, no sign of any deficits; Mac would be fine.

I am grateful and blessed to have the opportunity to work in a profession where miracles do happen.

Mac discharged to home with his mom and dad, a happy, healthy five-year-old!

## My Seasons

The stars are my springtime,
Dancing so high.
The stars are my springtime,
On a deep velvet sky.
The stars are my springtime,
Shining silvery and high.
But what if the stars should all flicker and die?
What then, my friend? What then?

The wind is my summer,
So blue and so pure.
The wind is my summer,
A time of great cure.
The wind is my summer,
So free and so gay.
But what if the wind should
Stop blowing one day?
What then, my friend? What then?

The sun is my autumn,
So golden and bright.
The sun is my autumn,
When birds take their flight.
The wind is my autumn,
Bringing all sweet, warm light.
But what if the great sun
Should stop in its flight?
What then, my friend? What then?

—AW

SUSANLEE WISOTZKEY

*The sky is my winter,*
*So gray and so deep.*
*The sky is my winter,*
*When all things must sleep.*
*The sky is my winter,*
*But when it all melts*
*And I hear the rain falling*
*In small, little pelts,*
*What then, my friend? What then?*

*—AW*

# CHAPTER 7

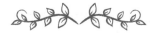

*Katrina (name's changed for privacy)*

This is a story told by a new nurse I had the pleasure to meet. Linda relayed this story and the positive effect it had on not only her patient but also the other staff members in her hospital.

For many years, the policy on our acute psychiatric ward was that patients could not go outside. This was primarily due to lack of or ability to create outside space within the organization and safety issues with patients attempting to elope. With the closing of state-funded psychiatric facilities, we had begun to see longer and longer length of stay for psychiatric patients. Staff and patients felt dissatisfied about the fact that patients could not go outside and get some fresh air. Acute psychiatric hospitals were for acute stabilization, medication management and transfer to lower level of care, or discharge to outpatient treatment. The acute psychiatric hospitals were not set up or equipped to care for patients on a long-term basis.

This hospital had an enclosed outside terrace with a beautiful garden area, a perfect place to take patients. It was outdoors, yet it would provide structure so that the patients could have a safe place to go outside, to breathe fresh air, and to feel the sun. The policy for taking patients outside was revisited to address the long-stay patients. The result, the creation of a new policy, which received approval.

The outcome of this policy for this institution was the overall positive effect on the geriatric and depressed patient population.

Linda relayed her wonderful experience, stating, "I had the opportunity to observe Katrina while she was sitting outside in the meditation garden. Her facial expression said it all. She was grinning from ear to ear, her eyes closed, and her face was to the sun. There was a peace about her. She was taking in the sights and sounds around her. She pointed out trees and flowers and identified them by name. She commented on the heavenly breeze and the birds chirping around us. We discussed our favorite seasons and driving in the car with the windows down. I felt privileged to be a part of that moment with Katrina, to see the joy and happiness she experienced with things most of us take for granted on a daily basis—fresh air, sunshine, birds. She reminded me that each day is a gift, which we should embrace and see with a fresh set of eyes."

How can you help a woman who is mentally impacted by her physical deformity that, when she is required to be out of her room, she covers her entire body with a blanket so people cannot see her disfigurement, so people do not stare? How do you, as the primary caretaker, stand apart from other hesitant hospital employees and provide her the care she deserves? Linda said, "Think outside the box or, rather, outside of the hospital."

Katrina was a young woman who first suffered from quadriplegia several years ago and then was a victim of a fire that burned a large percentage of her head, chest, and arms. She had extensive skin grafts, which were removed from parts of her that were tattooed, so she was a patchwork of very pale skin, tattooed words, and bright-red burn areas. She only had about 40 percent of her head hair, and she kept her head shaved to eliminate one spectacle.

Linda described how she paid close attention to Katrina's routine. Every day she was in bed and refusing breakfast until her bed bath at 9:30 a.m. She transferred to a lounge chair after her daily bath and breakfast. She was wheeled to the open milieu in the TV room, where she tried to be invisible on the periphery with the blanket pulled over her head. At 11:30 a.m., she ate lunch with assistance and stayed covered in the milieu until 1:30 p.m., when she requested to go back to her bed. That was where she remained until nine thirty the next morning and the process started over.

Linda spoke to how she started thinking about ways to break up Katrina's severe monotony of her current circumstances. Linda discovered Katrina loves baths. Katrina stated, "They cheer me up." Could Katrina have a bath? The unit had a lift. Linda took the initiative to see if the lift would work, dragging it down the hallway into Katrina's room and attempting to squeeze it through the tub room door, but the lift would not fit through the door.

"I love going out on beautiful days," Katrina shared. When was the last time Katrina was outside? She had been in this hospital for five months. Linda went into her room and asked her if she would like to go outside. Katrina was very tentative in her answer: "Do you think that would be okay with the doctor?" Linda told her she would try to get an order from her doctor to take her out into our atrium.

The following day, I had the order, and I was very excited for her to be taking her out. I was a new nurse, in orientation on my new unit, and I was considered an extra hand on the floor. I told her I was going to be taking her outside, and I expected her to pull the blanket over her head so that employees and visitors would not be able to gawk. She left the blanket down and paid attention to all the details while I was wheeling her through all the corridors.

We finally reached our destination on a perfect spring day. It was sunny and seventy-six degrees outside. The breeze was blowing, and the flowers were in full bloom. We parked in the shade, and I asked Katrina, "When was the last time you were outside?" "I can't remember," she said. Then she said something that broke my heart. She said, "How long do we have?" "We have as long as you want," I said. This was the benefit of being an extra hand on the floor; I could grant her this luxury.

Her facial expression said it all; she was grinning from ear to ear. There was clearly a peace about her. She said that she loved listening to the birds. I had not even noticed them. She was able to point out the trees and flowers and identify them by name. We were quiet most of the time, just people watching, feeling the heavenly breeze, and soaking up the sunlight. I asked her if she wanted me to uncover her toes so that she could wiggle her toes in the breeze—a guilty pleasure of mine. She said that she didn't think other people would want to look at her feet. After most of the people out returned to work, I uncovered her feet, and she wiggled her toes. She said, "That's all the more that I can move them." I responded, "What you can do is great!"

I was privileged to be part of that moment with Katrina. What she gave me on that one day was a gift of a lifetime. On this day, Christine *is* Katrina's nurse.

*"Each day is a gift which we should embrace and see with a fresh set of eyes."*

## Constant Motion

*She loved to see the bright lights flashing,*
*To speed along with never braking.*
*She loved the sounds of crowds and cities,*
*Hear laughter, anger, people faking,*

*To fly along the highway, doing sixty-five,*
*If not spinning wheels, a dead man alive,*
*Catch the wind in golden threads,*
*Weaving it away again in music.*

*I taste the dust and feel the rain,*
*As towns roll past, to slip away.*
*The sound of tires squealing,*
*A world revolves, goes reeling.*
*Constant motion,*
*To sense the commotion,*
*Slow, slow…*
*Stop.*

*—AW*

CHAPTER 8

## Long Road

I am hoping that this short grouping has given you a glimpse of the depth of the heart behind the nurse who cares for you or a loved one.

Nursing is a rewarding, challenging, and exhausting profession. It comes from the soul of your very being.

Each day, new nurses leave our profession, and older nurses retire. I wanted to give a quick look at what makes a nurse a nurse so others can understand the compassion, heartache, passion, dedication, sacrifices, and miracles that take place in the life of a nurse.

May God bless you with a compassionate nurse to provide care to you or the ones you love.

Stay safe, be happy, and wash your hands. ☺

# ABOUT THE AUTHOR

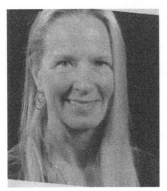 Dr. Susanlee Wisotzkey is director of neuropsychiatry at UCI Health and received a BA in psychology from Farleigh Dickinson University in Rutherford, New Jersey; a BSN from York College of Pennsylvania; a MSHSA from University of Saint Francis, Joliet, Illinois; and a PhD in health administration from Kennedy Western University. Dr. Wisotzkey has presented nationally and internationally on the topic of tight glucose control in the Roux-en-Y gastric bypass patient, presented and published on nurse retention, creating serenity space and medication safety. She is a past president of the Eta Eta Chapter of Sigma Theta Tau International Nursing Honor Society. She is a member of and volunteers for numerous organizations and nonprofits. Her residence is located in Pennsylvania, but she tirelessly works in Orange County, California. But above all, she loves being a registered nurse.

CPSIA information can be obtained
at www.ICGtesting.com
Printed in the USA
LVHW091131080221
678693LV00004B/395

9 781662 414183